Last Will and Testament

According to the Divine Rites of the Drug Cocaine

Scott Shaw

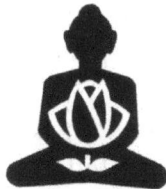

Buddha Rose Publications

First Edition 1988
Second Edition 2011

ISBN 10: 1877792004
ISBN 13: 978-1877792007

10 9 8 7 6 5 4 3 2 1
Printed in the United States of America

Last Will
and Testament

*According to the Divine Rites
of the Drug Cocaine*

Introduction

Sometimes the world pounds down hard on you and illusion offers a far better alternative to the hell granted by the mundane/by the alone. So, you move out into that promised land from which you may never return.

If drugs are so bad, then why do they make you feel so good? So good until you take that one-step out over the edge, where your grasp on reality is shaky and your ability to remain alive is completely removed from your control. That is what this text is about: that desire of illusion, that one step out over the edge; that place where experience is gained, realizations are had, enlightenment is known, and death may inadvertently become your only friend.

1

almost forgot about my tape
recorder
twelfth of June
just about 1:31 A.M.

I might die tonight
I am, I am fucking way too high
I did way too much coke but...
if I do go
I want no one to cry any tears over
me
because then I will be free

I have a certain remorse
about my lack of accomplishment
musically, literarily, artistically
but, I hope no one cries any tears
over me

I am walking on the pier right now
I am going to talk in a few minutes
if I make it

(my breath is shallow)

walking down Pier Avenue, now

past the bars
trying to grasp onto a bit of reality
my heart is like, is like
hurts weird

people coming so…

Hermosa Avenue now
turning to just walk down by the
bars
then I'll go back down to *The
Strand*

oh, my heart hurts
and I am fighting for air

for awhile when I…
the reason I keep stopping
is my mouth is so dry
it's funny there was a soda machine
but I didn't have any change

I keep licking my lips
but …
I keep feeling like I am going to
pass out
and now I'm feeling like

I'm going to do it again

funny, in my observation notebook
I kept writing
a whole bunch of observations
about a cocaine high
and this is the one place not to get
to
where you're going to die
and I...
if I have a heart attack...
what have you...

(cough)

I initially thought to return home
just after about a block of walking
on *The Strand*

(deep exhale)

hard to breathe

because I wanted to ditch my coke
in...
If I went down

that way I wouldn't/couldn't
get arrested for at least that...

because I have a lot of coke at
home

so I don't know if walking is good
for me
I think it is
it kind of keeps my system
working, you know but talking and
walking
it is hard for me to concentrate...
on breathing, and so...

(laughter)

I have never been this high
actually my feeling is pretty gro-o-
o-o

(end of side of tape)

had to turn the tape over

(deep exhale)

actually my feeling,
as I was saying, is pretty grounded
but my body is breaking down

(deep exhale)

so I'm going to stop talking now
and concentrate on breathing
I don't know whether it's a good
idea
to go home and take a valium or
not
could be though
could be
I'll have to think

(burp)

cocaine burp
and I've been drinking all this java
tonight
funny, I wanted to…

trying to get some liquid to
swallow
nada there

nada
nada
nada

but it's funny
I wanted to like

start pushing myself to start
staying up later again
four or five in the A.M.
so I could get creative
and start working on the books
in the night
like I like to do

    I've been fighting the
remaining
    last journey to Asia
    jetlag

so I drank some steamed *espresso*
two giant cups of it
and that stuff usually puts me up,
you know, till the early morning
hours
one cup usually does
but because of my...
still not complete adjustment
to the time zone...

there are some people though...
OK
kinda past
what was I saying
awh, about the coffee, you know,
and the time zone

so I wanted to start staying up later
and getting creative
to alleviate my artistic frustration
but...

may have done one notch too many

interestingly enough what I did
see what I did
what I did was bang down
two very heavy lines
just before I left
because I had come down,
you know, to a reasonable level
and awh...
then I had to have that typical
cocaine
go back and do one more thAng
that one more line

so I went and dug my stuff out
where I stash it
in the drawer
and chopped up
another couple lines

and I banged 'em
they were heavy back up lines

and I think that...
you know...
because I was down
but I'm still very high
I've been snorting coke all night
    all day and all night

but I didn't have the high feeling

    (deep exhale)

and so awh...
that's what did it
is that, that awh,
last minute quarter gram
that I put up my nose

probably did down about a gram-
ski tonight
maybe more
maybe plus
maybe gram-ski plus

funny, here comes a bicycle rider
so I'm going to chill for a second

cocaine comes on

he just rode by but...

14

cocaine, you know it's that
that waiting for the high
but then when it hits
it's a BAP!

but you know the feeling is
is that lying promise

    I will never do this again
    if I live through it

but awh...
you know, it's interesting
observations
I really don't have an addictive
desire to this drug
but it's more like an experiential
type thing
it's like
why not go ahead and do it
you know, get that kind of head
and get the distance to where...
if I don't create
I don't hate myself

    (deep exhale)

etc.

let's see what it does

I get periodic dizzy spells
I'm walking here...

so I guess I said all there is to say,
awh

I believe I'll make it
and I believe I'll do cocaine again
but I should set down, seeeet
doooown
some kind of definition to myself
because I'm not the young man I
once was
you know
although, I'm not old,
I guess twenty-nine, coming up fast
on thirty
but um...
my heart is not that great

(deep exhale)

it has always given me bits of
problems
here and...

I feel real dizzy right now

I feel really high

there's somebody up there, but
um…

I, I hope the walking has helped me
I think it must for it gets my system
circulating

then I got to go home and drink
some…
water
a lot of it
no more *java* though, not this
evening

but if I live through this
the experience will be well worth it
and as I'm saying
I'll probably do it again
but hopefully with someone else
this time
because, you know…
this is just no good alone
to get in this position where
nobody's there
to dump your coke for you
to keep you from the arm's of the
law

and take you to the hospital
if you need to go

I think it's really bad
there's somebody out on their patio
I think they just walked in

it's almost summer
although it's cool tonight

a lot of people out in the late night

it's now...
about 1:41 A.M.

god, it seems a lot longer than just
ten minutes
when I said it was, 1:31

god, I almost went out/passed out
I got to, to grab reality
I can't let myself slip

   (deep exhale)

god, I'm really wa... way wasted
my head is spinning right now
I can't let myself go down

it was worse though
when I first started out
well, no
I think this is about
this is about equal

it's the talking
I should breathe better

I'm going to leave the tape on just
in case
I go down,
but ... as I say
if I die
then I'll be free

don't cry no tears over me

(deep gasp)

(steps, steps, steps)

(deep gasp, for air)

this is about as
worse as it's been
with this spinning
head
it's not spinning
but I just feel like

I'm going to pass out any second

(step, step, step)

(deep gasp)

(step, step, step)

some more of it must have hit my
system
through my nose or whatever

(step, step, step)

it's hard to concentrate on
breathing

my heart is just like...
feeling really weird

my hands are getting numb

Oh shit!

(deep exhale)

it's like as I started out
there is a part of me
that wants to stop
but there is a part of me

that has to get home

maybe I over exerted myself, I
don't know

I walked kinda fast, I think

I feel like... (unrecognizable word)

(step, step, step)

it's nothing just now
it's like when I walked out, I uh...

and when all this shit started hitting
me
just it's like when I walked around
the building I was just high...
then the minute I hit *The Strand*
it was like over-powering
and 1 almost went down

(cough)

and it was like uh, unconscious,
I sniffed in really deep
and I thought
shit, I took in too much more of
this shit

I got to quit doing it now
so I tried to pick my nose clean a
little bit

(burp)

awh, cocaine burp
this is definitely the highest I have
ever been physically
not mentally

(step, step, step)

I guess this is like Japan
and the poems I wrote that drunken
night

it's funny my business manager
kept,
keeps saying
what a fiasco that trip was for me
financially
but it produced a book of poetry

so few ever understand art
how could that have bad?
no matter what the cost…

maybe this will be my last will and testament

(step, step, step)

(deep exhale)

(step, step, step)

(exhale)

(step, step, step)

a bicycle just went by

(step, step, step)

(unrecognizable ramblings)

(deep exhale)

I've never been so high like this before...

(step, step, step)

(sniff)

(step, step, step)

(exhale)

(step, step, step)

almost at the end of *The Strand*
here
one more block

(deep exhale)

(vague talking by other
people)

shit, two people just startled me
I hope that doesn't do in my heart

that adrenal rush

I don't know
it is really going to my head
my heart now

(exhale)

walking back down and around
to Hermosa Avenue now

my heart hurts

hard to breathe

(talking by other people)

the thing about valium is
I don't want to mix up drugs in
my system
too much like that
take me down and out
I don't know

guess I'm just going to have to
wait this out

I don't know

almost home

so I'm signing off here
I guess what comes, is what comes
and what ever does is all my fault
but...
as I say, if I die
at least I'll be free

interestingly enough my head
doesn't even feel high
though I suppose

(cough)

in retrospect I will think that I was
but I don't feel it

ah life
what a dance

[taken from the tape,
verbatim]

2

home
alive or dead
well, that is always a narrow
margin
T.V. on
take my mind
take it from the pain
to the pain
take it anywhere
but where I am

3

2:00 A.M.
telephone call
the answering machine
2:03 A.M.
"Well, fuck that, she must be
home."
"I think I will try again."

"Hello."
"Hello."
"Oh, it's you."
"How are you my L.A. Scottish
prince?"
"Dying."
"Did a bit too much cocaine."

      her story is lost
      as this semi-fine
      sweet young white bread
      type of thing, be

      crazy
      yeah, way over the deep end
      and I do mean literally
      not figuratively

It was S.F.
(San Francisco), for the
uninitiated
a few days before
at an exhibit opening
she stared deeply into the lost
realms
of some painting
that only she could see

personally, truthfully
I thought that she was *dupped*
up on some Acid with that
distant and dilated
look in her eyes

well hey
I can play along

so we stared together
for an hour or so
then the museum closed
we were out-a-there
a walk on *the Streets of San
Francisco*

like the T.V. show
remember?

then a bar

she had *dos* Singapore Slings

(don't get me thinking of
Asia)

me, I had *uno* mineral water

we then exchanged
in the magic of the moment
the most perfect first kiss of
my life
then to her crib
then to a semi-serious sex
session

"How's Mr. Cat?"
"You mean Muffy?"
"Whatever."

her fucking cat
spent the night
that night
the night I spent with her
continually waking me up
by trying to sleep on my face

as I told him

I was seriously thinking
of finding some hungry
Vietnamese
in the area

"Oh, he's fine."
"He misses you."

in the morning, I awoke

(with the little sleep which I
actually had due to all the
ongoing/on-feeling sex)

to, how shall I say
a rude awakening

her eyes
were just as distant
and her words
as tilted as the night before

anyway,
her insanity didn't bother me
as much
as the violence she dished out
when I tried to bail
I mean real
Play Misty for Me

Clint Eastwood action

but that is all in some other
piece of literature
in some book
unwritten/not completed

in my vast library of things to
do...

(A long story, made very
short).

never will I see her again
never, never, never.

but then...
somewhere
in this lost cocaine O.D.
session
somehow I felt a calling
a calling to call her
to make promises in the night
to know that there is willing
love waiting

I had received, that day,
Monday
two, count them two

lost love letters from her

oh yeah, I had taken my
Uncle Scotty's advice,
        "Love them and leave
'em
        and don't give them
        your phone number."

thus the letters

"Will you come and see me? I need
you. I want
        you. I love you."
"Yes, tomorrow. If I'm still alive. I
will come
        tomorrow. I will fly up there.
I will rent
        a car. We will be together. I
don't care if
        you're crazy."
"Good night"
well alright

a moment lost from the pounding of
my heart
the knots which it was trying to
form

though my breath was short
periodic rushes to the brain
and a wonder
as to whether

I would indeed be alive

manana
If so, I had a date

  A date I never kept
  letters that continue to come
  which I never answer

dead or alive
life is all perception

in her mind
which am I

I really don't even care

4

T.V.
douses my mind
I flip through
the cable sent channels

a moment of this
a second of that
bad movies
bad T. V. shows
they all have become so
predictable
they all have become so boring

5

my heart
it is alive
alive, on its own
"IT'S ALIVE!"
I want to scream
I, on the other hand,
am in perpetual question

6

Do I say, "Never again?"
like on one of those
one too many
wake up in the morning
hangover sessions
no
I do not
alive or dead
what a way to go
hold the art tight
hold it with a reason
hold it with a vengeance
and die
in its artistic arms

O.D.
or suicide
a far better way to go
than at the hands
of some foolish
disease
that you have no control over

    (a disease like age)

7

3:00 A.M.
time to talk again
give me a reason
to hold on to reality
telephone in hand
dial the number
three rings
and *nada*

my sweet little
Japanese
former rich girl
former babe
now a bit overweight
nuisance
who calls me and calls me
twice, three times a day
every day
wanting a date
but no, I want a dream
not a date
and one worth living
one worth feeling
one worth taking a chance with and
for
but now

now...
you can serve a purpose
a purpose past the one you served
upon our meeting
what was it,
yes, three years ago

no answer
no purpose
you served nothing

three rings
I know you are home
but I do not wish
to wake your aging parents
so three rings is it
bye-bye
to a hello
which 1 never received

8

life
its destiny
its call
it definitely
called me out tonight

9

am I alive
am I dying
well, in truth
who can ever really say
who ever really know

my heart
yes, my heart, it still knots
my breath
well, I am breathing
my head
down for hours or more

cocaine
the goddess
cocaine
the life
and how it slips out of our grasp
so easily
I love it

I love to feel /I love to live

just sometimes
I wish that living
felt a wee bit better

10

three hours
passed and plus the walk
alive?
well, more or less

I'm going to live
live through it
this time anyway

the light is coming out
coming up

I guess I will go to bed

11

5:45 A. M.
my telephone rings
international call
I hear the static
on the line

"Malaysia calling Dr. Scott Shaw."
"Yes."
"Is this Dr. Scott Shaw?"
"Yes."
"Malaysia calling."

    a bit redundant there,
    aren't you babe

"Hello Scott... Hello..."
"Yes."

    now to shorten the convo
    and the statement of fact
    it was my babe
    one of my babes
    K. L.
    (Kuala Lumpur, for the
    uninitiated)
    on the line

from the line
Malaysia
it had been two weeks
since I was there
since I saw her last

"My sister is dying of cancer."
"Then she will be free."
"How can you say that, Scott?"
"She had it and never told anyone."
"Be happy for her. She'll be free."
"How, can you say that, just how can
you say that?"
"Because I am here dying. Dying
from too much cocaine. I want no
one to cry any tears over me. I want
them to be happy."
"You can't die! I love you Scott."
"So."
"All my friends say that I'm a fool.
They tell me you have women all
over the world. They tell me you
say, *I love you,* to all of them.
They tell me to forget you."
"They are right."

        now to abbreviate a half hour
        plus convo

into its shortest possible
application
she *rap'd* on about her sister
I told her there was nothing
that she could do
she was worried about me
I told her if I died
to be happy because then I
would be free

"Bye, bye."

I had hung up
before she had the opportunity
to sufficiently, (to her standards)
tell me how worried she was of and
for me

I tried to chill back
and catch some Z's

RING!

"Malaysia calling Dr. Scott Shaw."
"Yes."
"Is this Dr. Scott Shaw?"
"Yes."

good, she wasn't redundant
this time

"Scott! are you OK?"
"Just see me in the wind."

as I hung up
I could hear her scream

"WAIT!"

play it
play it full on
live it
bring the melodrama to life
breathe it
to the maximum

and finally I went to sleep

12

I definitely cracked a piston on this
one
well, I have cracked them before
the only problem is
that I do not have many more to
crack
before it is down for the count

not the standing eight
like this sweet session

but down for the big one
ten on the canvas

so I say,
dream on dreamers

live on

feel on

whatever the price is
pay it

for living empty
with no experience to show for it

is a far worse fate
than to die at the hands
of a momentary high

13

Last Will and Testament

and to you I leave
my bad little '64 Porsche 356 SC
I always promised it to you anyway
it has a personality crisis at the
moment
it is still in the shop
so you, you can pick up the tab

and I leave to you my guitar
collection
do what you must
do what you will with it/with them
but remember they are all works of
art
and most you will never see again

and I leave you all of my paintings
the ones I did
the ones you did
even the ones I have purchased
for who else do I know
who else have I ever known
that would/that could
ever appreciate art

as you have/as you do

as well, I leave you all my poetry
and all of my other written works
including my journals

please try to understand the space I
was in
when I wrote many of the things
that I said

I guess that's it
I guess I leave you everything
no one else even matters
no one else ever has

I leave you everything
everything but my debts
them, I cast to the realms
of the checked out
dying and dead of unpaid,
no way to collect
never-never-land
bye-bye-ville
to the credit card companies
unpaid, dollars lost forever, bills

but all else
my cameras

my bicycles
my library
my records, CD's, etc.

all to you
for who else has ever known me
better
who else has known me more
all to you
my main L.A. Babe
my forever L.A. Lady
who I have not even seen
in such a long time
the joke is
I do not even know where you are
we have lost each other in the
wind
the winds of time
the winds of change
but I will leave that to the
attorneys
that's the gift
I leave to them
to find you
and give you all my worldly
possessions
wherever it is
that you may be
whatever it is

that they may be worth

and mostly I give you
an eternal loving kiss, goodbye
and a sorry for all the hell
I put your through
a sorry for the me, being me
you were too good
to have lived through that
the me, being me
hopefully this will pay you back
in some small way

14

as the seventh day
comes to a close
I am still not
one-hundred percent on
this bad boy
definitely did
take me for a ride

a knot in my heart
here or there

a day or two of separated and
spaced vision

> but distance is a dream
> a dream to the underachieved
> distance holds a key
> unlocking the necessity
> to not accomplish anything
>
> my journey jetlag
> is curing
> my heart, well...
> it probably will heal
>
> and the session

now it is
for the record
for the fools like I
who find poetry in the wind
and experience
at the gates of death

dream on...

seven days later and I'm still
alive...

S.
88.27.6
Redondo Beach, California